I0436718

Copyright

Copyright © 2015 by C. H. Truelove.

Disclaimer

Although every precaution has been taken to verify the accuracy of the information contained herein, the author and publisher assume no responsibility for any errors or omissions. No liability is assumed for damages that may result from the use of information contained within.

This book is not intended as a substitute for the medical advice of physicians. The reader should regularly consult a physician in matters relating to his/her health and particularly with respect to any symptoms that may require diagnosis or medical attention.

Table of Contents

Introduction

If there's one thing I've learned over the years caring for sick patents is that being sick is emotionally difficult and mind numbing. It can be very scary for most people. Your mind and your health are the greatest gifts in life. So, don't let illness take away your hopes and dreams. You were placed on this earth for a reason, and that reason doesn't stop until you do. No matter what your situation, you have a contribution to make.

The mind is a powerful instrument. It can change everything in your life for the better, but it can also change things for the worse. Having a positive attitude can have a huge impact on your life and your overall health.

Spend more time with your friends and family or go on a walk with the dog, and if you don't have a dog get one. Having a dog or cat can have a positive influence on your health by reducing stress. Therapy dogs visit at the hospital for this very reason. Positive beliefs and keeping a positive attitude can really make you feel better and have a lasting effect on your life in general.

Your life is a mission from God. Don't let illness change your mission or keep you from being who you were put on this earth to be.

> *"Beliefs have the power to create and the power to destroy. Human beings have the awesome ability to take any experience of their lives and create a meaning that disempowers them or one that can literally save their lives."*

Anthony Robbins

With that said……….Let's get started!

Living with Congestive Heart Failure

Imagine waking up one morning and it feels like a tight band is around your chest. You feel like you are unable to get enough oxygen into your lungs. Your anxiety level goes all the way up to the ceiling and you sit up abruptly think, what is going on? You know you haven't felt the best lately, but this is scary.

Or, what if you have several errands you need to run around town, but first you want to go to the mailbox and get the mail. As you are walking to the mailbox, you get short of breath and find that you are suddenly very tired.

Maybe you sit down to rest and see that your ankles and feet are swollen and when you touch them, your fingers leave indents in the skin that stay a few minutes after you take your hand away. Or, you notice that even though you are not eating more than usually, your clothes feel tighter around your waist.

This is what a person living with Congestive Heart Failure (CHF) deals with on a daily basis when the condition is not under good control. According to the American Heart Association, uncontrolled CHF is responsible for over 1 million hospitalizations each year. The economic impact of this condition hurts both your wallet and the health care system's bottom line. This book will assist you in gaining control over your CHF and help you to live a healthier, active life with CHF.

What is CHF?

To combat CHF and understand why and how it happens, we first need to get to know our heart – its purpose, its function, and how to keep it healthy.

There is a Glossary in the back of this book to help you better understand some of the medical terms used within. Pictures and diagrams are used as well to assist with understanding some medical concepts.

The heart is an amazing muscle that works as a pump continuously moving blood to vital organs in the body. When that pump loses its ability to function efficiently the rest of the body can suffer due to the decrease in oxygen-rich blood. This condition is called CHF.

The heart's pumping mechanism is impaired when its muscles become inflexible or bulky, which decreases the chamber's ability to constrict or pump. CHF also can occur when one or more of the chambers of the heart becomes enlarged and is unable to pump blood effectively. When the heart cannot pump the correct volume of blood through its chambers, it causes fluid to back-up and congestion occurs.

This process starts a chain reaction of events that include not enough oxygen reaching the kidneys, which slows down production of the urine that would normally relieve the body of excess sodium. The congestion is caused by blood pooling as well as excess sodium retaining fluids in surrounding tissue.

The congestion can occur in either the venous system that is returning blood to the heart or the pulmonary system, depending on which side of the heart is failing.

The left side of the heart pumps oxygen-rich blood through the arteries to the rest of the body. When that side's lower chambers, known as the ventricles, are damaged, the blood backs up into the lungs and causes shortness of breath or difficulty breathing. This is known as left-sided heart failure. It can also lead to a decrease of oxygenated blood to the rest of the body including the kidneys, which can lead to multiple systems to fail.

Right-sided heart failure is most commonly caused by left-sided heart failure. The right side of the heart receives venous (oxygen depleted) blood returning from the rest of the body. When the right side of the heart is not working, the fluid congestion is usually in the abdomen and lower legs.

There is no cure for CHF – no magic pill or procedure that will instantly relieve the associated pain, nor the damage it does to your body. Left untreated, CHF's effects on your body can be devastating. Fortunately there are lifestyle changes that you can implement to help protect your heart from further damage and gain control over your CHF to live a healthier life with a noticeable improvement in quality of life.

Causes of CHF

There are many causes of CHF. The most common is Coronary Artery Disease (CAD), also known as atherosclerosis. This is the process of plaque build-up in the coronary arteries that narrow the vessels and reduce blood flow to the heart muscles. Much like on your teeth, plaque is a detrimental substance that is directly related to the foods we eat.

This build-up can lead to a heart attack, which is scientifically termed a Myocardial Infarction (MI). The plaque build-up narrows the arteries that feed the heart muscles, eventually becoming partially or completely blocked. When this happens, the part of the heart that was getting blood supply from that artery sees its function greatly reduced or severely damaged.

Another cause of CHF is hypertension (HTN), more commonly known as high blood pressure. The high pressure of blood flowing through the heart causes the heart to work harder. This, like any exercise of any muscle in the body, causes the muscle to enlarge or bulk up and become less efficient.

Damaged heart valves can contribute to CHF. Valves that are stretched out can cause blood to flow backwards or stagnate in a chamber of the heart. This backflow makes the heart work harder and can lead to the formation of a blood clot. If the blood clot travels through the bloodstream to the lungs, heart or brain, it can be fatal. Constriction of a heart valve reduces the amount of blood that can be pushed through the opening and increases the workload of the heart.

Other causes of CHF are chronic drug and alcohol use. The toll that drugs in general, and cocaine specifically, places on the heart can lead to heart muscle damage and failure. Cocaine speeds up the heart rate and over time can enlarge the heart. Intravenous (IV) drug use is known for causing infections that attach themselves to the heart valves. Chronic alcohol use results in increased fluid intake and poor nutrition which can result in heart failure.

Unfortunately, there can be idiopathic or unknown reasons for CHF. CHF is usually a secondary condition caused by other cardiac issues. Other chronic medical conditions such as anemia, sepsis (system-wide infection), Chronic Obstructive Pulmonary Disease (COPD), diabetes and renal failure can contribute to CHF.

Medications That Treat CHF

The good news is that in today's medical world, there are many medical treatments to help with CHF. By establishing and maintaining an effective treatment plan with your cardiologist, the prognosis and the chance of leading a normal active life increase dramatically.

There is a wide and varied array of medications that can assist the heart to improve function. Medications are placed in categories that are determined by their purpose. We will look at these categories and their role in CHF. This list is to help you get familiar with the different classes of medications and their uses. New medications come on the market daily, so be aware that this list may not be all inclusive. Your best bet to stay current on medical research is to have regular consults with your cardiologist and primary care doctor. To keep up with the latest news on CHF, visit websites like the American Heart Association, which is dedicated to dispersing the latest information on heart disease and heart care.

Anti-hypertensives – can work in several different ways but the end result is the same, to decrease the pressure of blood in the vessels and heart. There are several classes of anti-hypertensive medications.

> • Angiotensin is produced naturally by the body and raises blood pressure by causing blood vessels to constrict. An *Angiotensin-Converting Enzyme Inhibitor* (ACE) will often

be used to prevent the body from making angiotensin. If this fails to reduce blood pressure by itself, *Angiotensin Receptor Blockers* (ARBs) can be added to further reduce the amount of angiotensin in the body. Your doctor also may use vasodilators such as *Nitroglycerin* for better blood pressure control.

- *Digoxin* may be used to strengthen the force of the heart's contraction to help push blood throughout the body. Beta-Blockers are beneficial to slow your heart rate down if the heart is in a tachycardic (fast) rhythm and to improve heart muscle strength. When blood pressure is controlled, blood flows freely and the load of work on the heart decreases dramatically.

There can be negative side-effects such as blood pressure dropping too low or a dry cough. Be sure to monitor your blood pressure regularly and discuss possible side-effects with your doctor.

Blood Thinners – can help in two ways. First, they decrease the viscosity (thickness) of the blood so it can travel more easily throughout the body and heart. Another use is to decrease the blood's ability to clump and by doing so, reduces the chance of blood clot formation. Some of these medications have been on the market for years and require frequent blood testing to ensure therapeutic levels are achieved.

Blood that becomes too thin can lead to dangerous problems with bleeding. Newer medications coming on the market have lower risks of bleeding and do not require frequent lab work.

Diuretics – also known as a water-pill, work in conjunction with the kidneys and excrete excessive water and sodium out of the body through urine. Potassium sparing diuretics and loop diuretics do similar tasks, but without affecting your potassium level as much. These medications can be used together to increase effectiveness.

Potassium – is a natural mineral that the body produces to help keep the body's electrolytes in balance. One function of potassium is muscle contractibility, so if the level of potassium is out of range, either high or low, it can affect heart contraction which can lead to abnormal heart rhythm. Another possible symptom of low potassium is muscle cramps. Because sodium and potassium work together to keep balance in the body, once sodium is targeted to be excreted, so is potassium. A potassium supplement is used to replace what the diuretics removed.

Oxygen – may be needed at times to supplement your oxygen supply when your condition is aggravated by circumstances.

Regardless of what prescriptions your cardiologist ends up recommending, the most important thing to remember is that medications only work when they are taken. Follow the instructions given by your doctor and don't stop or skip any medication without first consulting with him or her. If you have any concerns or questions about how to take a medication or what the side-effects can be, talk to your doctor or pharmacist. Make sure to refill your medications early so that you eliminate the possibility of running out, especially when planning for a trip or vacation. Medications can help tremendously with gaining control over CHF, but they can't do it alone. Lifestyle changes, even small ones, can increase your chances of living an improved life with CHF.

10 Simple Steps to Take Control of Your CHF

1. Weigh Yourself

Weigh yourself daily at approximately the same time of day, such as first thing in the morning, after you urinate and before you eat. Use the same scale each time you weigh. Also, be aware of the amount of clothes you are wearing when you weigh. Keep this consistent so that you are able to detect any weight change. If you notice a weight gain of two pounds in a five-day period, call your doctor. This could be an early sign of fluid building up in your body. The doctor might change your medication regimen to compensate for the fluid build-up. Likewise, be on the look-out for other signs of fluid build-up such as lower leg swelling, clothes fitting tighter around the waist or increase in shortness of breath.

Write your results down to look for increases in weight, and to document your weight for your next doctor visit. Keeping track of your blood pressure and heart rate might help your doctor create a good treatment plan. There are modern options available for blood pressure cuffs that may be covered by your healthcare plan. These machines are quick and accurate to measure you blood pressure on a daily basis. By arming yourself with the knowledge of your daily weights and blood pressure readings, you can give your doctor an amazing amount of information so that he or she can help you succeed in the long term.

2. Diet

One of the quickest ways to make progress in taking control of your CHF is to make changes in your diet. To begin with set small goals that will be easy to accomplish in a short period of time. The benefit of completing these achievable goals is positive feedback and will keep you on track for positive results.

The most important goal is to decrease the amount of sodium (salt) in your diet. The aim is to keep your sodium intake below two grams a day. If you are a visual person this may help, a single salt packet from your favorite take-out/fast food restaurant is approximately one gram of sodium. Also, look carefully at processed food labels for sodium content. Beware of foods that claim to be low-fat, as while they may have fat removed, it's at the expense of a large infusion of sodium to give flavor to the product.

Adding foods that are a good source of potassium to your diet help to counteract the effects of diuretics. You might be taking a potassium supplement but natural selections are better. Sources of potassium include

- sweet potatoes
- squash
- tomatoes

- beans

- yogurt

- milk

- bananas

- fish

- soy beans

Adding heart healthy foods such as whole grain, nuts, fresh fruits and fresh vegetables to your diet is an important goal. Substitute whole grain for refined grains in products such as bread, rice and cereal. Whole grains are high in fiber and natural nutrients such as the B vitamins, magnesium and folic acid that can increase your heart's health. Aim for three 1 ounce servings a day. By using fresh fruits and vegetable instead of canned fruits or vegetables, you can decrease the amount of sodium as well as gain natural nutrients that have a positive effect on your heart and health. Eat 4-5 servings of both fruits and vegetables each day. Try substituting fish and lean meats for that have marble like fat throughout. Use fat-free or low-fat dairy products. Fiber can lower risks for heart disease and can curb your appetite. Increase your intake to equal 20-30 grams a day.

Altering the way you cook food is an essential goal for a healthy heart. Use baking or grilling as an alternative to frying. Steam your fresh vegetables instead of using canned vegetables. Other healthy methods of cooking include roasting, broiling, poaching and stir-fry. When using oils to cook, go for oils like olive oil or canola oil instead of oils that have trans-fats or saturated fats. Trans-fat comes from commercially friend or baked goods such as doughnuts and cookies, as well as home shortening that is solid, not liquid. Saturated fat comes from animal products like bacon and lard. It can also come from some vegetables such as cocoa butter, palm oil and coconut oil. Be sure to remove the skin from poultry before cooking as well as excess fat on red meat. Also skim fats off of stews and soups before serving or freezing.

Another goal is to regulate fluid intake. This has to be done carefully. You do not want to overload yourself with fluids that will be difficult for your body to remove. But on the flip side, you don't want to take in too little fluid and become dehydrated. Ask your doctor what a good daily fluid intake would be for you. A good way to keep track of what you drink is to use a container that has measurements on the side and write down ALL fluids that you ingest. This includes food items that melt into fluids such as ice, ice cream and Jell-O.

While you are attaining the goals above you will also reduce your caloric intake. Reducing your caloric intake coupled with increasing your exercise will result in weight loss. There are several apps to help you keep track of your ratio of calorie intake and exercise to optimize your weight loss. If you are not into technology, keeping a diary of your calorie intake is simple. To lose weight, you need to take in fewer calories than you expend.

> **Rule of thumb:** Men burn approximately 15 times their body weight in pounds a day. Women burn about 14 times their body weight in pounds a day. EX: Man weighs 200 pounds (200 x 15) expends 3,000 calories a day. He will need to either decrease his caloric intake to around 2,500 calories a day or exercise to expend more calories.

3. Exercise

Establish a daily exercise routine such as walking. You don't have to hike for hours, just 30 minutes a day will help to improve circulation in your entire body. Work up to the 30-minute goal in small intervals by starting with five minutes a day. Before you start, use an extended warm-up routine to naturally dilate vessels before moving into exercise. Walking also assists blood return to the heart by activating small valves in the legs to push the blood back up to the heart. This lowers the risk of blood clots formation because of blood pooling in the lower legs. Rest when you need to and if at any time you experience a significant increase in shortness of breath or severe tiredness, stop exercising and call your doctor. Yoga, swimming or resistance training can also be beneficial for people with CHF. **Consult**

with your doctor before starting any exercise regime.

4. STOP Smoking

Nicotine can produce serious problems for people with CHF. Nicotine increases your heart rate and constricts blood vessels, which leads to increases in blood pressure. People who smoke have a tendency for clumping of blood and blood clots. Smoking also has a negative impact on the lungs and reduces oxygen levels throughout the body. **STOP SMOKING** - this allows the blood vessels to relax and remain open which permits blood to flow freely.

5. Relaxation

It is necessary for your body and heart to have significant time to rest. While at rest, the heart can more easily pump blood throughout the body. If your lower legs have swelling, be sure to elevate them while resting to assist your heart's functionality. Recently, the amount of quality sleep you get has been found to be tied to heart health. Low quality sleep has been linked with heart disease which can cause CHF. Sleep can be difficult to come by if you have a busy life with multiple commitments such as family and work, but you must consider your own health as a top priority. Getting 7-8 hours of sleep consistently is the best way to ensure your body has enough time to rest between active cycles. While some people are able to function on considerably less sleep, their quality of life and health suffer as a result.

Meditation has been used successfully to achieve lower blood pressure, decrease heart rate, lower stress levels and increase lung capacity. There are several types of meditation, so choose one that is right for you and reap the rewards. Just 20-30 minutes a day can improve the health of your heart, body and mind.

6. What You Wear

Wear loose fitting or non-restrictive clothing to increase your blood flow throughout the body. Clothes that bind or are too tight can cause resistance in blood flow and make the heart work harder. Stockings or socks that cut into the leg or ankle can increase pooling of fluid in lower legs, ankles and feet. Your doctor may suggest compression stockings/socks, to help reduce fluid retention in lower legs. Measurements will need to be done to ensure an accurate fit and reduce the possibility of restricting blood flow.

7. Avoid Extreme Temperatures

Extreme hot or cold temperatures can increase the work load of the heart by trying to regulate the body's core temperature. Be sure to dress appropriately for the weather and be cautious in extreme situations. Take precautions to keep your body at the appropriate temperature. If it is HOT outside – stay indoors where there is air conditioning, avoid caffeine and alcohol. If the weather is COLD – layer clothes and wear mittens or gloves and a hat.

8. Immunizations

Keep up-to-date on immunizations such as flu and pneumonia. Both of these infections are lung related and can decrease oxygen levels, which in turn places an extra burden on the heart. Also avoid large crowds during cold and flu season and stay away from people you know are sick.

9. Keep Your Own Medical Record

Have an accurate and up-to-date list of your medications. Include medications that have been prescribed by your doctor and any vitamins or supplements that you take as well. This is to reduce the risk of interactions between medications that can cause harm to you. Also keep an up-to-date list of any procedures or surgeries you have had done. When you first have a procedure or surgery, you think you will never forget when I had this done, but over the years, memories fade – write it down. A good idea is to keep these records on your computer then print it out so that you may take it with you when to go for a doctor's visit or are admitted to a hospital. Also take it with you when you go on a road trip or vacation. You never know when something unexpected will happen.

10. Collaborate With Your Doctor(s)

A good, trusting relationship with your doctor(s) is invaluable. If multiple doctors are involved in your care due to other medical conditions, be sure to have a complete and accurate list of your current medications for each visit. This will ensure that your medications will work with each other instead of causing more harm than good. Make sure you keep your appointments and actively participate in your care. Keeping other medical conditions under control and by working closely with your doctor, you can avoid many issues that can derail your chance of taking control of your CHF.

When to Seek Help

It is important to know when you should seek help. Here are some pointers to look for:

Call your doctor if you have:

- Weight gain of 2-5 pounds in a 5-day period.

- Increased shortness of breath or wheezing.

- Unusual tiredness/fatigue or inability to complete normal tasks.

- Increased coughing, especially with activity.

- Difficulty sleeping or lying flat in bed.

- Noticed swelling in hands, feet, ankles, legs, abdomen.

- Acceleration in heart rate or palpations.

- Dizziness or lightheadedness upon standing.

Seek immediate help if you experience:

- Difficulty breathing.

- Mental status changes like unable to focus or decreased alertness.

- Chest pain or discomfort.

- Fainting.

Glossary

Arteries – blood vessels that distribute oxygen-rich blood to the body and organs.

Atrium – one of two upper chambers of the four chambers in the heart.

Cardiologist – a physician that specializes in the study of the heart.

Coronary Arteries – supplies blood directly to the heart muscles.

Electrolyte – a substance that, in fluid, conducts an electric current. Acids, bases and salts are an example of electrolytes found in the blood stream.

Potassium – an electrolyte in the body that works with sodium to keep many bodily functions in balance.

Primary Care Physician – a physician that specializes in general practice such as Family Practice or Internal Medicine.

Prognosis – prediction of the course of a disease or condition, estimation on chance of recovery.

Pulmonary System – the lungs and vessels that oxygenate blood.

Sodium – an electrolyte in the body that helps to maintain a healthy balance. Also can be known as common table salt.

Venous System – blood vessels that return oxygen depleted blood from the body to the heart and lungs for re-oxygenation.

Ventricle – one of two lower chambers of the four chambers in the heart.

About The Author

C. H. Truelove – Registered Nurse with a Bachelor of Science in Nursing – understands the importance and benefits of having tools to help achieve a healthy lifestyle. Her passion in the healthcare field, and in particular cardiology, has led her to reach out to others, through written word and blogging, to help them gain the tools they need to improve their overall health and well-being.

With more than 24 years working in the healthcare field and 8 years specializing in heart related conditions, she was motivated to pursue one of her goals to put her specialized knowledge of cardiac medicine to print. By becoming an author, online publisher and blogger, she can reach a wider audience and assist more individuals in their quest for a healthier heart.

Thank You!

Thank you so much for purchasing this book!

My hope is that this book will give you accurate information on Congestive Heart Failure and steps to make to improve your life with CHF. As you take the steps suggested in this book, you will see a noticeable difference.

By taking control of your Congestive Heart Failure you will be able to live a more active and healthier life.

Lastly, if you have enjoyed this book, **please leave a review on Amazon on the product page where you purchased this book.** This kind act will help me to reach more people.

Thank you and good luck with your journey to better health.

But wait! There's more!

You can visit my Website

www.SoundHeartToday.com

There are articles, exercises and heart healthy recipes that will enhance your chances of succeeding in your quest to better health while living with CHF.